Chair Yoga For Weight Loss

A Comprehensive Guide to Chair Yoga Transformation: 28 Days to Balance, Flexibility, and Weight Loss

By

Anthony D. Anderson

Table of Contents

Introduction

Welcome to "Chair Yoga for Weight Loss: A Comprehensive Guide to Chair Yoga Transformation: 28 Days to Balance, Flexibility, and Weight Loss!" In the pages that follow, we're about to embark on a remarkable adventure—one that promises to reshape your body, cultivate balance, and set you on the path to achieving your weight loss goals. The best part? You can do it all right from your favorite chair.

In today's hectic world, finding the time and space for traditional workouts can feel like an insurmountable challenge. But fear not, because Chair Yoga is here to revolutionize your fitness journey. It's a gentle, yet incredibly effective practice that adapts the ancient wisdom of yoga to a seated setting, making it accessible to all.

Over the next 28 days, we'll guide you through a carefully crafted program that's tailored to meet you wherever you are on your fitness journey. Whether you're a complete novice or someone looking to take their yoga practice to the next level, we've got you covered.

Week 1: Building the Foundation is your starting point. We'll gently introduce you to the basics of Chair Yoga with soothing stretches, mindful breathing exercises, and a touch of mindfulness. This week, you'll begin to experience the joy of increased mobility and the peace of a quieter mind.

Week 2: Gaining Momentum is where the magic truly begins. As you become more comfortable, we'll introduce you to increasingly advanced chair yoga poses and help you strengthen your core. Our daily motivation and mindfulness tips will ensure you stay focused and inspired.

Week 3: Embracing Challenges is where you'll discover your hidden potential. Get ready to tackle advanced Chair Yoga routines that will push your boundaries, enhancing not only your balance but also your flexibility. We'll address those moments when you feel stuck and provide self-care strategies to keep you moving forward.

Week 4: The Final Push marks the climax of our journey. We'll guide you through high-intensity chair yoga routines designed to accelerate your weight loss journey. As you look back on the incredible progress you've made, you'll be amazed at what's possible.

In our conclusion, we'll celebrate success stories and urge you to make Chair Yoga a lifelong practice. This guide is about so much more than just shedding pounds; it's about reclaiming your body's potential, discovering newfound balance, and nurturing your overall well-being. Throughout these pages, you'll find detailed 28-day guided exercises, nutritional wisdom to complement your chair yoga practice and additional resources to fuel your curiosity. A transforming journey awaits you, are you prepared? The chair is your throne, and your body is your vessel. Let's begin this remarkable 28-day Chair Yoga adventure together!

Chapter 1

The concept of Chair Yoga

In the world of fitness and well-being, Chair Yoga stands out as a unique and accessible practice. In this discussion, we'll explore the essence of Chair Yoga, and specifically, how it can be an effective and gentle approach to weight loss. Let's dive into this concept using simple and easy-to-understand language.

Understanding Chair Yoga

Chair Yoga is a specialized form of yoga that adapts traditional yoga postures for individuals who may have physical limitations or prefer a gentler approach to exercise. Instead of complex floor poses, Chair Yoga uses a chair for support, making it an inclusive practice suitable for people of various ages and fitness levels.

Why Choose Chair Yoga for Weight Loss?

At first glance, you might question how sitting in a chair can assist in weight loss. It's a reasonable question. While Chair Yoga might not have you breaking a sweat like an intense workout, it offers a range of benefits that can contribute to weight loss in a gentle and sustainable way.

1. Improved Metabolism: Chair Yoga involves gentle movements and stretching, which can help enhance your metabolism over time. A well-functioning metabolism is crucial for burning calories and assisting with weight loss.

2. Enhanced Muscle Tone: Regular Chair Yoga practice engages different muscle groups, leading to improved muscle tone. It's important to note that muscles burn more calories than fat, which is a positive factor when aiming for weight loss.

3. Mindful Eating: Chair Yoga often includes mindfulness techniques and controlled breathing. These practices can help you become more aware of your eating habits. Mindful eating may prevent overindulgence and encourage healthier food choices.

4. Stress Reduction: Emotional eating and weight gain are two consequences of stress.. Chair Yoga incorporates relaxation and stress-reduction techniques that can help you manage stress more effectively, potentially reducing the urge to snack on unhealthy foods.

5. Balanced Hormones: Some Chair Yoga poses have a positive impact on the endocrine system, aiding in the regulation of hormones that influence your appetite and metabolism.

Incorporating Chair Yoga into Your Weight Loss Journey

Chair Yoga is adaptable for people of all fitness levels, making it suitable for beginners and those with physical limitations. You can start with simple poses and gradually progress as your strength and flexibility improve. Consistency is key to experiencing the benefits of Chair Yoga for weight loss.

In conclusion, Chair Yoga might not resemble your traditional weight loss regimen, but its gentle and accessible nature makes it an invaluable tool for your journey. The combination of increased metabolism, muscle tone, and mindfulness can contribute to shedding those extra pounds and achieving a healthier lifestyle. So, take a seat, grab a chair, and embark on your Chair Yoga for weight loss journey today.

Setting the stage for a 28-day transformation journey

Are you prepared to take the first steps toward improving your health? Chair Yoga, a gentle and accessible practice, can be your trusted companion on this path to weight loss. In this comprehensive discussion, we'll walk you through the process of setting the stage for a 28-day transformation journey with Chair Yoga, all explained in simple and easily understandable language.

Start with Simplicity

We understand that starting a weight loss journey can be daunting, but with Chair Yoga, it's remarkably simple. You don't need to be an expert in fitness or yoga. This practice meets you where you are, regardless of your age or fitness level. Whether you're a beginner or have physical limitations, Chair Yoga can be tailored to your unique needs.

Daily Dedication

Your first step on this journey is committing to a daily practice. Consistency is the key to reaping the benefits of Chair Yoga for weight loss. By dedicating a small portion of your day to a Chair Yoga session, you create a calming and rejuvenating routine that sets a positive tone for the rest of your day.

Structured Progression

Over the next 28 days, you'll progressively move through a structured program of Chair Yoga. Each day introduces you to different poses and exercises, building on your previous practice. This gradual progression aims to enhance your strength, flexibility, and overall well-being in a safe and sustainable manner.

Nutritional Guidance

In addition to the physical aspect, your transformation journey includes a focus on nutrition. Understanding what you eat and how it affects your body is crucial for your weight loss goals.

The program provides simple and practical nutritional tips that complement your Chair Yoga practice. It's not about restrictive diets but making informed and mindful choices.

Mindfulness and Emotional Balance

Weight loss isn't just about physical changes; it also involves your mental and emotional well-being. Chair Yoga incorporates mindfulness and relaxation techniques that can help you manage stress, stay focused on your goals, and foster a positive relationship with your body.

Supportive Community

You don't have to go on this adventure all alone. There are Chair Yoga communities and resources available online and locally. Connecting with others who share similar goals can provide encouragement and motivation throughout your journey.

Celebrating Progress

As you progress through the 28 days, it's essential to celebrate your achievements, no matter how small they may seem. Weight loss journeys have their ups and downs, and it's crucial to acknowledge your successes, no matter how modest. Every step you take in the right direction is a victory.

In conclusion, setting the stage for your 28-day transformation journey with Chair Yoga is a manageable and inclusive process. With daily dedication, structured progression, mindful nutrition, and a supportive community, you're well on your way to achieving your weight loss goals. So, are you ready to embrace this remarkable journey, take a seat, and let Chair Yoga guide you toward a healthier and happier you?

Chapter 2: Week 1 - Building the Foundation

Welcome to the next step in your Chair Yoga journey for weight loss. Before we dive into the daily routines and exercises, it's crucial to start by "Building the Foundation." This subchapter lays the groundwork for a successful 28-day transformation. Here, we'll focus on creating a supportive environment, setting achievable goals, and understanding the basic principles of Chair Yoga. By building this foundation, you'll be well-prepared to make the most of your weight loss journey. So, let's get started and set the stage for a healthier you.

Day 1-3: Chair Yoga Basics for Beginners

Congratulations on taking the first step in your 28-day journey with Chair Yoga for weight loss! These initial days are all about building a strong foundation, just like you'd start learning the basics of anything new. In this section, we're going to guide you through Day 1 to Day 3, focusing on Chair Yoga basics designed especially for beginners.

Day 1: Getting Comfortable

On your first day, we want you to get comfortable with the idea of Chair Yoga. Sit down in a sturdy chair, one without wheels, and find a quiet space where you can relax. This is your personal yoga haven. Begin with simple stretches – reach up to the sky, gently twist your torso, and flex your toes. Breathe deeply and feel your body starting to awaken.

Day 2: Breathing and Relaxation

Day 2 is all about the breath. Chair Yoga places a strong emphasis on controlled breathing, which helps calm your mind and increase awareness. Practice simple breathing exercises: inhale slowly through your nose, and exhale through your mouth. It's like taking a moment to pause and recharge, preparing your mind for the journey ahead.

Day 3: Introduction to Mindfulness

Now, let's explore mindfulness. Mindfulness is all about being present in the moment, fully aware of your thoughts and sensations. Sit on your chair comfortably with your eyes closed, and take a few deep breaths. As you inhale, imagine breathing in positive energy, and as you exhale, release any stress or tension. It refreshes your mind.

Remember, these first three days are your building blocks, your solid foundation. Take your time and don't rush. Feel the energy and strength that comes from within, just like the roots of a tree grounding it firmly. Your Chair Yoga journey is just beginning, and we're here to support and guide you every step of the way. So, are you ready to embrace the basics and set the stage for your transformation? Let's begin!

Gentle stretches and breathing exercises

As we continue with our foundation-building in these early days, it's all about gentle stretches and breathing exercises. Let's dive right in and make these practices a part of your daily routine.

Day 1: Gentle Stretches

Today, we focus on gentle stretches. Think of your body like a rubber band. Stretching it carefully is essential to prevent injury and increase flexibility. Begin by sitting comfortably in your chair. Extend your arms overhead, lengthen your spine, and feel the gentle stretch from your fingers to your toes. Take your time, and remember to breathe steadily as you stretch. It's like greeting the day with a smile, slowly waking up your body.

Day 2: The Power of Breathing

Now, let's explore the power of breathing. Breathing is your body's built-in stress buster. Sit back in your chair and take a deep breath in through your nose, allowing your abdomen to rise. Exhale slowly through your mouth, letting the tension slip away. Breathing exercises are like a mini-vacation for your mind, giving you a sense of peace and calm.

Day 3: Harmonizing Body and Breath

Today, we bring it all together by harmonizing your body and breath. Start with gentle stretches, and as you stretch, inhale deeply. As you release the stretch, exhale slowly. This synchrony between body and breath is like a beautiful dance, promoting relaxation and inner harmony.

As you practice these exercises in these early days, you're beginning to build a solid foundation for your Chair Yoga journey. Like constructing a house, each brick plays a vital role in the final structure. You're strengthening your body, calming your mind, and setting the stage for a healthier, more vibrant you.

So, are you ready to continue these gentle stretches and breathing exercises? Let's keep the momentum going as we move forward in our 28-day transformation journey.

Introduction to mindfulness

In your Chair Yoga journey for weight loss, we've already embarked on gentle stretches and breathing exercises. Now, let's take a closer look at "Introduction to mindfulness." It's a powerful tool that can make a significant difference in your well-being and weight loss.

What is Mindfulness?

Being fully aware of the current moment is what mindfulness means. It's about paying full attention to what's happening right now. It's like giving yourself a break from the constant whirlwind of thoughts and worries that can sometimes fill your mind.

Why is Mindfulness Important?

Mindfulness has numerous benefits. For one, it helps reduce stress. Imagine a calm lake with no ripples – that's the kind of serenity you can find through mindfulness. It can also boost your mood, enhance your focus, and improve your overall quality of life.

Practicing Mindfulness

To practice mindfulness, no special training or equipment is needed. You can do it anywhere, anytime, even while sitting in your chair. Here's how to get started:

1. Find a Quiet Spot: Sit in a comfortable chair in a quiet place where you won't be disturbed.

2. Close Your Eyes: Gently close your eyes to help shut out distractions.

3. Breathe: Take a few deep breaths to calm your mind. Feel your breath as you inhale and exhale.

4. Observe Sensations: Pay attention to the physical sensations in your body. What do you feel? Any tension or relaxation?

5. Acknowledge Thoughts: Thoughts may pop up; that's okay. Just notice them without judgment and let them pass like clouds in the sky.

6. Stay in the Moment: Focus on your breath and the sensations in your body. Stay in this moment for a short while.

Mindfulness and Weight Loss

You might wonder, how does mindfulness relate to weight loss? Well, it can be a game-changer. Mindful eating, for example, is about paying close attention to what you eat, savoring each bite, and recognizing when you're full. This can lead to better food choices and prevent overeating.

So, practicing mindfulness can help you stay more in tune with your body and emotions, making it an essential part of your Chair Yoga journey. It's like having a secret weapon in your pocket, supporting your goals and making your journey enjoyable and meaningful.

Are you ready to introduce mindfulness into your daily routine? Let's continue on this path, making small but powerful changes along the way.

Day 4-7: Increasing Mobility

As we move forward on your Chair Yoga journey for weight loss, we're diving into the days dedicated to "Increasing Mobility." This phase is like building the road that will lead you to a stronger and more flexible body. So, let's get started!

Day 4: Embrace Mobility

On Day 4, it's time to embrace mobility. Start by sitting in your chair, and gently move your arms in a circular motion. This exercise may seem simple, but it's a fantastic way to wake up your joints and improve your range of motion.

Day 5: Stretch and Lengthen

Now, let's focus on stretching and lengthening your body. Sit back in your chair, and slowly extend one leg in front of you, then the other. Sensate the stretch in your calves and hamstrings. This is like stretching the canvas before painting a beautiful picture. Your body gets ready for what's about to come.

Day 6: Building Strength

Day 6 is all about building strength. In your chair, do seated leg lifts. One leg should be raised and held for a short while before being lowered. Repeat on the other side. This exercise helps strengthen your legs and core, making you more stable. Consider it as setting the building blocks for a solid foundation.

Day 7: Balance Enhancement

Balancing is crucial to mobility. Practice lifting one foot slightly off the ground while seated. Hold it for a moment, then switch to the other foot. This simple exercise improves your balance, which is like adding the finishing touches to a masterpiece.

By the end of these four days, you'll notice improved mobility and flexibility. Your body will feel more responsive, like a well-tuned instrument. Plus, increasing mobility can help you perform more complex Chair Yoga poses as you progress in your 28-day journey.

So, are you ready to take these steps towards increased mobility? Keep in mind that every day you're getting closer to your weight loss goals. With each exercise, you're building a body that's more capable, more flexible, and more resilient. Let's keep the momentum going!

Beginner-level chair yoga poses

Now that you've established your foundation and increased your mobility, it's time to explore "Beginner-Level Chair Yoga Poses." These poses are like the building blocks of your Chair Yoga practice, helping you to improve strength, flexibility, and overall well-being on your weight loss journey. Let's delve into these beginner poses step by step.

Pose 1: Seated Mountain Pose

- Your feet should be placed flat on the floor while you sit comfortably in your chair.
- Stretch your back and let your shoulders relax.
- Inhale, raising your arms overhead.
- Exhale, bringing your hands to your heart center.
- This pose is like grounding yourself, feeling strong and steady.

Pose 2: Seated Forward Bend

- Begin in a seated posture while keeping your feet flat on the floor.

- Inhale and lengthen your spine.

- Exhale, hinging at your hips, and reach for your toes.

- Hold for a few breaths, feeling the stretch in your back and hamstrings.

- It's like a gentle morning stretch, helping you awaken and feel more flexible.

Pose 3: Seated Cat-Cow Stretch

- Sit comfortably while placing your hands on your knees.

- Inhale, arch your back, and lift your chin (Cow Pose).

- Breathe out, curve your spine, and bring your chin toward your chest (Cat Pose).

- Repeat this flowing motion several times.

- It's like a gentle massage for your spine, keeping it flexible.

Pose 4: Seated Spinal Twist

- Sit with your feet flat, and cross your right ankle over your left knee.

- Inhale, lengthen your spine.

- Exhale, gently twist your torso to the right.

- Hold for a few breaths, feeling the twist in your spine.

- This pose is like wringing out stress and tension from your body.

Pose 5: Seated Knee Lifts

- Sit in your chair while your feet are flat.

- Inhale, and lift your right knee towards your chest.

- Exhale, lower your foot.

- Repeat on both sides.

- This workout helps to make your legs stronger.

These beginner-level chair yoga poses are your stepping stones to a more flexible and stronger body. Think of them as the foundation of your practice, just like building a house from the ground up. They provide you with the strength and stability you need to continue on your weight loss journey with confidence.

So, are you ready to start practicing these beginner-level poses? Remember, consistency and patience are your allies. With each pose, you're progressing toward your goals. Let's keep moving forward!

Incorporating balance-enhancing routines

In your Chair Yoga journey for weight loss, we've explored beginner-level poses that build strength and flexibility. Now, let's focus on "Incorporating Balance-Enhancing Routines." Balance is a key component of a healthy body, and it's a vital element in your weight loss journey. So, let's dive into these routines that will help you find your center and improve your overall well-being.

Routine 1: Seated Leg Lifts

- Your feet should be placed flat on the floor while you sit comfortably in your chair.
- Inhale and lift your right leg, keeping it extended.
- Hold for a short while before lowering your foot.
- Repeat with your left leg.
- This exercise helps you work on your leg strength and balance.

Routine 2: Seated Knee to Chest

- Begin in a seated posture while keeping your feet flat on the floor.
- Inhale, and as you exhale, bring your right knee to your chest.
- Hold for a few breaths.
- Lower your foot and switch to the left knee.

- This routine aids in improving your balance and mobility.

Routine 3: Seated Ankle Circles

- Sit in your chair, and extend your legs.
- Lift your right foot, and begin making circles with your ankle.
- Repeat in both directions.
- Switch to your left ankle.
- Ankle circles help improve ankle stability and balance.

Routine 4: Seated Tree Pose

- Begin in a seated position.
- Raise your right foot to rest on your inner thigh on the left.
- Hold your hands in a prayer position in front of your heart.
- Hold for a few breaths.
- Repeat with your left foot.
- This pose promotes balance and concentration.

Routine 5: Seated Warrior I

- Sit with your feet flat, right knee bent, and left leg extended.
- Inhale, raise your arms overhead.
- Exhale and turn your torso toward the right knee.
- Hold for a few breaths, feeling the stretch.
- This routine builds core strength and balance.

Incorporating these balance-enhancing routines into your Chair Yoga practice is like adding layers of stability to your weight loss journey. It's akin to placing bricks that make your journey smoother and more secure.

So, are you ready to incorporate these routines and enhance your balance? Remember, every small step you take in these routines contributes to your overall strength and well-being. Keep moving forward with determination and patience. Your weight loss goals are well within reach!

Daily tips for staying motivated and mindful

On your 28-day journey with Chair Yoga for weight loss, motivation and mindfulness are your companions for success. These daily tips are like your guiding stars, helping you stay on track and making your journey more enjoyable and meaningful.

Tip 1: Set Realistic Goals

Start with achievable goals. Instead of focusing on a big weight loss number, think about small, consistent changes. These small victories will keep you motivated.

Tip 2: Celebrate Progress

Enjoy the moment every day that you've made progress. Whether it's mastering a new pose or simply showing up on your mat, acknowledge your efforts. This positive reinforcement is like a pat on the back, boosting your motivation.

Tip 3: Practice Mindful Eating

Mindful eating means savoring every bite, paying attention to your body's hunger cues, and avoiding distractions while eating. It's like turning your meals into a mini-meditation, helping you make healthier food choices.

Tip 4: Stay Consistent

Consistency is key. Make Chair Yoga a daily habit. Whether it's a 5-minute routine or a full session, the more you practice, the more you'll progress. It's like watering a plant every day – it grows stronger with regular care.

Tip 5: Find Your Support System

Consider joining a Chair Yoga community or partnering up with a friend. Sharing your journey and goals with others can provide valuable support and motivation. It's like having cheerleaders in the stands, urging you on.

Tip 6: Embrace Mindfulness

Mindfulness isn't just for yoga; you can incorporate it into your daily life. Take a moment to pause and breathe. It's like hitting the refresh button for your mind, keeping you present and focused.

Tip 7: Enjoy the Journey

Lastly, remember to enjoy the journey. It's not just about reaching your weight loss goal; it's about the experience along the way. Find joy in each pose, each breath, and each moment of mindfulness. It's like savoring the beauty of a scenic route, making the journey as delightful as the destination.

These daily tips are here to support you throughout your Chair Yoga journey. They are like the wind beneath your wings, helping you soar towards your weight loss goals with motivation and mindfulness. So, are you ready to embrace these tips and make each day a step towards a healthier, happier you? Keep going, and remember that you've got this!

Chapter 3: Week 2 - Gaining Momentum

Welcome to Week 2 of your Chair Yoga journey for weight loss! You've already laid the foundation, increased your mobility, and explored beginner-level poses. Now, it's time to dive deeper into "Gaining Momentum." Just like a snowball rolling down a hill, we're picking up speed on your path to a healthier you.

Building on Progress

In Week 1, you set the stage for your transformation. You became familiar with the basics of Chair Yoga and started your journey towards increased flexibility and balance. Week 2 is all about building on that progress. Think of it as moving from the first few chapters of a book to the exciting middle, where the story really starts to unfold.

Challenging Yourself

As you delve deeper into Chair Yoga, you'll encounter new poses and routines that might be more challenging. But remember, challenge is where growth happens. These challenges are like the turning points in your favorite adventure story, pushing you to become stronger and more resilient.

Increasing Intensity

In this week, you'll also notice an increase in intensity. Your practice might become a bit more demanding, just like the rising action in a movie that keeps you engaged. It's all part of your journey towards a healthier, happier you.

Staying Mindful and Motivated

Throughout Week 2, the daily tips for staying mindful and motivated will continue to be your companions. They're like the reassuring voice of a trusted friend, reminding you to celebrate your progress, set achievable goals, and practice mindfulness, both on and off the mat.

Your Chair Yoga Adventure Continues

So, are you ready to continue your Chair Yoga adventure in Week 2? We've already taken the first steps, and now we're gaining momentum, just like a river flowing steadily towards the sea. Each day brings new challenges and new triumphs, and you're writing your own success story. Stay motivated, stay mindful, and let's keep moving forward towards your weight loss goals. Week 2 awaits, and you're well on your way to becoming the best version of yourself. Let's do this!

Day 8-14: Progressing Towards Intermediate

As you enter the second week of your Chair Yoga journey for weight loss, you're well on your way to building strength, flexibility, and overall well-being. Now, it's time to take the next step and delve into "Day 8-14: Progressing Towards Intermediate." Just like a story that gains depth and complexity, your journey is evolving.

Day 8: Exploring Intermediate Poses

On Day 8, you'll start exploring intermediate poses. These are like the advanced chapters of your Chair Yoga book. Don't be intimidated; they're designed to challenge and empower you. You'll find that with consistent practice, what seems complex today will become accessible tomorrow.

Day 9: Deeper Stretches and Balance

Day 9 is about deeper stretches and balance. You'll feel your body reaching new heights of flexibility. Just like a skilled tightrope walker, you'll find your balance and grace, and with every pose, you'll notice a growing sense of control.

Day 10: Incorporating Flow

It's time to incorporate a flow. Flow is like the rhythm of a dance – smooth and graceful. As you move from one pose to another with grace and intention, you'll enhance the fluidity of your movements, strengthening both body and mind.

Day 11: Mindfulness in Motion

Mindfulness is not just about stillness; it's also about being mindful in motion. You'll practice being present in every move, just like an artist painting a masterpiece, each stroke deliberate and meaningful.

Day 12: Embracing Challenges

Embrace challenges as opportunities for growth. When you face challenging poses, it's like overcoming obstacles in your journey. These challenges will be your stepping stones to success.

Day 13: Finding Inner Strength

Inner strength is your superpower. You'll discover that it's not just physical strength that matters but the resilience and determination that come from within. It's like unlocking a hidden treasure within yourself.

Day 14: Celebrating Progress

In Week 2, you'll continue to celebrate your progress. You gain momentum toward the weight loss goals you have everyday. These daily celebrations are like milestones that mark your path to success.

Progressing towards intermediate poses is an exciting phase of your Chair Yoga journey. It's like turning the page to a new chapter in your favorite book, where the plot thickens, and the adventure deepens. With each day, you're stepping into a stronger, more flexible, and more confident version of yourself.

Are you ready to embrace the challenges and the growth that Week 2 brings? Keep going, and remember that every pose you practice is a step towards your weight loss goals. Your Chair Yoga adventure is in full swing, and you're the hero of your story. Keep the momentum going!

Intensified chair yoga poses

In the second week of your Chair Yoga journey for weight loss, we're taking things up a notch as we explore "Intensified Chair Yoga Poses." Just like turning up the volume on your favorite song, these poses add intensity and energy to your practice, helping you build strength and flexibility.

Pose 1: Seated Forward Bend with Twist

- Sit with your feet flat and knees together.
- Inhale, lift your arms overhead.
- Exhale, bend at your hips, and twist to the right, reaching your left hand towards your right foot.
- Switch sides after a few breaths of holding.
- This pose is like ringing out any tension in your body, creating a sense of lightness.

Pose 2: Chair Warrior II

- Sit with your feet flat, right knee bent at a 90-degree angle, and left leg extended.
- Inhale and stretch your arms wide.
- Exhale, turning your torso to the right.
- Hold for a few breaths, feeling the strength in your legs.
- This pose empowers you, like a warrior ready for action.

Pose 3: Seated Pigeon Pose

- Sit with your feet flat, right ankle on your left knee.
- Inhale, lengthen your spine.
- Exhale and then lightly press down on your right knee.
- Hold for a few breaths, feeling the stretch in your hip.
- This pose is like opening a door to deeper flexibility and freedom of movement.

Pose 4: Seated Boat Pose

- Sit with your feet flat, knees bent, and hands on your knees.
- Inhale and lift your feet off the floor.
- Balance on your sit bones.
- Hold for a few breaths.
- This pose strengthens your core, just like a sailboat navigating through waters.

Pose 5: Seated Mountain Pose Variation

- Sit with your feet flat and arms by your sides.
- Inhale, lift your arms to the sides and overhead.
- Exhale, bringing your hands together.
- Hold for a few breaths.
- This pose is like embracing the strength of a mountain.

Intensified Chair Yoga poses are your next step in this incredible journey. They bring a fresh challenge to your practice, just like hiking up a steeper mountain trail. With each pose, you're becoming more resilient, both in body and mind.

Are you ready to intensify your practice? Remember that with each challenging pose, you're progressing towards your weight loss goals. Keep your determination high and your spirit even higher as you continue this empowering journey. You've got this!

Focus on core strength

In your Chair Yoga journey for weight loss, one of the key areas to focus on is building core strength. Just like a strong foundation supports a house, a strong core supports your body. Let's explore the importance of core strength and some Chair Yoga exercises that can help you achieve it.

Why Core Strength Matters

Your core is not just about having a toned stomach; it plays a crucial role in your overall well-being. A strong core stabilizes your spine, improves posture, and enhances balance and coordination. It's like the anchor that keeps a ship steady in the storm.

Benefits of a Strong Core

1. Improved Posture: A strong core helps you maintain an upright posture, reducing strain on your back and neck.

2. Enhanced Balance: Core strength allows you to move with stability and confidence, reducing the risk of falls.

3. Better Mobility: With a strong core, you can move more freely and perform daily activities with ease.

4. Reduced Back Pain: Core exercises can alleviate lower back pain by providing support to the spine.

Chair Yoga for Core Strength

Here are some Chair Yoga exercises to help you focus on building core strength:

1. Seated Leg Lifts: Sit at the edge of your chair and lift your legs one at a time. This exercise engages your abdominal muscles.

2. Seated Bicycle Crunches: Sit with your hands behind your head and lift your knees, then bring your opposite elbow to your knee in a twisting motion.

3. Seated Boat Pose: Sit with your feet flat, lift your legs, and balance on your sit bones. This pose strengthens your core.

4. Seated Russian Twists: Sit with your feet flat, hold your hands together, and twist your torso to one side, then the other.

5. Seated Plank: Place your hands on the armrests, engage your core, and lift your body off the chair. This pose provides a strong core workout.

Remember, building core strength is a gradual process, much like constructing a sturdy bridge. Be patient and consistent in your practice, and over time, you'll notice increased stability and a stronger, more resilient core. Your core is the powerhouse that can help you achieve your weight loss goals, so keep focusing on strengthening it in your Chair Yoga practice.

Day 15: Midway Check-In

Congratulations on reaching the midpoint of your 28-day Chair Yoga journey for weight loss! As you enter Day 15, it's the perfect time for a "Midway Check-In." Just like taking a breather during a long hike to appreciate the view, let's pause and reflect on your progress so far.

Assessing Your Journey

By now, you've delved into Chair Yoga, built strength, increased mobility, explored various poses, and focused on core strength. It's like completing the initial chapters of a book, and now it's time to review what you've learned.

Celebrating Your Achievements

Take a moment to celebrate your achievements. Have you noticed increased flexibility, better posture, or a calmer mind? Celebrate these victories – they're like milestones on your journey.

Recognizing Challenges

During the first half of your journey, you may have encountered challenges. Whether it's the intensity of certain poses or simply finding time to practice, these challenges are like stepping stones to your personal growth.

Setting New Goals

Now, it's time to set new goals for the remaining days of your journey. What would you like to achieve by the end of these 28 days? Setting goals is like charting a course on a map; it gives you direction and purpose.

Rekindling Motivation

If you've hit a motivational dip, don't worry – it's normal. Use this check-in as a motivational boost. Let the reason you began this journey serve as your source of hope.

Sharing Your Experience

Consider sharing your journey with others. Whether it's with a friend, family member, or an online community, sharing your experiences can provide you with valuable support and encouragement.

Midway Reflection

In these first 15 days, you've laid the groundwork for a healthier, more balanced life. Think of it as reaching the middle of an exciting story, where the plot thickens, and the adventure becomes even more captivating.

So, as you embark on the second half of your Chair Yoga journey, remember that you're already well on your way to a healthier, happier you. Keep the momentum going, stay motivated, and savor each moment of your journey. Day 15 is just the beginning of the second act of your adventure, and the best is yet to come. Let's continue this incredible journey together!

Tracking progress and setting realistic goals

In your Chair Yoga journey for weight loss, tracking your progress and setting realistic goals are essential steps toward achieving your desired outcome. Just as a hiker uses markers on a trail to monitor their path, you, too, need a way to measure your success. Let's explore the importance of tracking progress and how to set achievable goals.

The Importance of Tracking Progress

1. Motivation: Tracking your progress is like having a cheerleader on your side. It can boost your motivation when you see how far you've come.

2. Accountability: It holds you accountable for your journey. Just as a diary records your experiences, tracking your yoga sessions and physical improvements keeps you responsible for your goals.

3. Feedback: It provides valuable feedback. You'll get insights into what's working and what might need adjustment, like a compass guiding you in the right direction.

How to Track Progress

1. Keep a Journal: Consider maintaining a Chair Yoga journal. Write down the poses you practice, how you felt during and after each session, and any improvements you've noticed.

2. Take Photos: Visual progress can be motivating. Periodically take photos of yourself to see physical changes over time.

3. Use Technology: There are many apps and fitness trackers that can help you log your Chair Yoga practice and monitor your progress.

Setting Realistic Goals

1. Specific: Goals should be clear and specific. Instead of saying, "I want to lose weight," you could say, "I aim to practice Chair Yoga for 30 minutes every day."

2. Measurable: Goals should be quantifiable. This way, you can measure your progress. For example, you could set a goal to increase your flexibility by touching your toes within a month.

3. Achievable: Make sure your goals are realistic and attainable. Setting small, achievable goals like practicing a new pose each week can build your confidence.

4. Relevant: Goals should be relevant to your overall objective. In your case, they should align with your weight loss journey.

5. Time-Bound: Give yourself a timeframe to accomplish your goals. For example, you could aim to lose a certain amount of weight in three months.

Setting realistic goals is like charting your course with a clear destination in mind. It keeps you focused and gives your efforts purpose.

Remember, your Chair Yoga journey is unique to you, and it's not about perfection; it's about progress. By tracking your progress and setting achievable goals, you're actively steering your path toward a healthier and happier you.

Daily tips for maintaining consistency and motivation

Consistency and motivation are like the fuel that keeps your Chair Yoga journey for weight loss running smoothly. To help you stay on track, here are some daily tips that will act as your guiding stars, making your journey more enjoyable and sustainable.

Tip 1: Create a Routine

Establishing a daily routine is like setting the stage for success. Choose a specific time each day for your Chair Yoga practice, and stick to it. Consistency becomes a habit when you have a routine.

Tip 2: Set Small Goals

Just as a staircase consists of individual steps, break your journey into smaller, achievable goals. Setting small milestones allows you to track your progress and celebrate your achievements.

Tip 3: Visualize Success

Take a moment to visualize your success. Imagine how you'll feel when you reach your weight loss goal. Visualization can be a powerful motivator, like seeing the finish line in a race.

Tip 4: Keep a Journal

Maintain a journal to record your daily progress. Write about your practice, how you felt, and any challenges you overcame. Journaling is like a map of your journey, helping you navigate your way to success.

Tip 5: Find an Accountability Partner

Sharing your journey with a friend or family member can provide motivation and accountability. Just as running buddies keep each other going, a partner can offer support and encouragement.

Tip 6: Embrace Variety

Variety keeps things interesting. Explore different Chair Yoga poses and routines to prevent boredom. Variety is like trying new flavors – it keeps your journey fresh and exciting.

Tip 7: Reward Yourself

Give yourself small rewards along the way. Reward yourself with something enjoyable whenever you've accomplished a goal. Rewards act as milestones and incentives for staying motivated.

Tip 8: Stay Mindful

Mindfulness isn't just about your practice; it's about being present in daily life. Practice mindfulness by being aware of your choices, especially in your eating habits. Mindful eating can help you make healthier choices.

Tip 9: Be Patient

Remember, progress takes time. Be patient with yourself. Just as a gardener nurtures a plant and watches it grow, your efforts will yield results with consistent care and patience.

Tip 10: Stay Positive

A positive mindset is like a tailwind that propels you forward. Focus on your achievements, no matter how small, and maintain a hopeful outlook. Positivity can overcome challenges.

These daily tips are your companions on your Chair Yoga journey for weight loss. They are like steady companions, guiding you with consistency and motivation. As you embrace these tips and make them part of your daily life, you'll find that your journey becomes more enjoyable, sustainable, and successful. Keep moving forward, and remember that you have the tools to achieve your weight loss goals. You're on the right path!

Chapter 4: Week 3 - Embracing Challenges

Welcome to Week 3 of your Chair Yoga journey for weight loss! As you enter this new chapter, we're shifting our focus to "Embracing Challenges." Think of this week as the turning point in your favorite novel where the characters face their greatest trials and emerge stronger. Your journey is taking on depth and complexity, and you're about to discover the heights of your own potential.

Rising to Challenges

Up until now, you've built a strong foundation, increased your mobility, and explored various poses. This week is all about rising to new challenges, just as heroes in an epic tale face formidable obstacles that test their mettle.

Pushing Your Limits

You'll encounter more demanding poses and routines that may seem daunting at first. Embracing these challenges is like scaling a mountain; each step takes you closer to the peak, where the view is breathtaking.

Building Resilience

Challenges are opportunities in disguise. They are like rainstorms that nourish the ground and make flowers bloom. By facing them head-on, you'll build resilience, both in body and spirit.

Deepening Your Practice

Your practice is deepening, like a river carving its path through rugged terrain. You'll notice that your poses become more precise, your breathing more controlled, and your mindfulness sharper.

Daily Tips for Guidance

Throughout Week 3, our daily tips will continue to be your trusted companions. They will provide guidance and encouragement as you tackle these challenges, much like a lighthouse guiding ships through rough waters.

Midway Check-In

Don't forget to reflect on your journey as we reach the midway point of your 28-day adventure. Just as characters in a story pause to reflect on their experiences, your midway check-in is an opportunity to celebrate your achievements, recognize your progress, and set new goals for the second half of your journey.

Stay Inspired

As you dive into Week 3, remember that every challenge you encounter is an opportunity to grow and evolve. Just like heroes in a legend, you have the strength within you to overcome obstacles and reach your goals. Stay inspired, stay focused, and keep your heart open to the adventures that lie ahead. Your Chair Yoga journey is a captivating story, and you're the resilient, determined protagonist. Let's keep turning the pages together!

Day 16-21: Advanced Chair Yoga

As you step into Days 16 to 21 of your Chair Yoga journey for weight loss, you're now exploring the realm of "Advanced Chair Yoga." Think of it as reaching the most thrilling part of your favorite adventure story, where the challenges are greater, but so are the rewards. These advanced poses will push your limits and help you grow both physically and mentally.

Day 16: Chair Yoga for Strength

On Day 16, you'll dive into poses that emphasize strength. These poses are like conquering a steep mountain trail, challenging but incredibly rewarding. You'll feel your muscles working, building power and endurance.

Day 17: Deepening Flexibility

Day 17 is all about deepening your flexibility. Just as a skilled painter uses finer brushes to add intricate details, you'll refine your movements and stretches. You'll notice your body becoming more supple and graceful.

Day 18: The Balancing Act

Day 18 is the balancing act. Advanced balancing poses are like walking a tightrope, demanding your full concentration. As you find your center and balance, your mind and body sync in a harmonious dance.

Day 19: Advanced Mindfulness

Mindfulness deepens on Day 19. It's not just about being aware of your body; it's about connecting with your inner self. These practices are like unlocking the deepest chambers of your heart and soul.

Day 20: Mastering Transitions

Day 20 is about mastering transitions. Just as a dancer glides between steps with grace and precision, you'll flow seamlessly from one pose to another. Your practice becomes fluid and seamless.

Day 21: The Culmination

On Day 21, you'll experience the culmination of your efforts. These poses are like the grand finale of a fireworks show – spectacular and awe-inspiring. You'll find strength, flexibility, balance, and mindfulness coming together in perfect harmony.

Advanced Chair Yoga is your next level, your final act, in this amazing journey. It's like reaching the climax of your favorite book, where all the storylines converge into one epic moment. With each advanced pose, you're growing stronger, more flexible, and more centered.

Are you ready to embrace the challenge of Advanced Chair Yoga? Keep in mind that every challenging pose is a stepping stone towards your weight loss goals. Your journey is a captivating adventure, and you are the brave, resilient hero. Keep moving forward, and relish the thrills of these advanced practices. You've got this!

Full-body workouts while seated

In your Chair Yoga journey for weight loss, you'll discover that seated workouts can be just as effective as traditional exercises, engaging your entire body while sitting comfortably. These exercises are like a hidden treasure chest, holding the key to a fitter, healthier you.

Why Full-Body Workouts Matter

Full-body workouts are like a symphony, where every instrument plays a crucial role in creating beautiful music. Engaging your whole body during your Chair Yoga practice has several benefits:

1. Efficiency: You're making the most of your time by working multiple muscle groups simultaneously.

2. Balance: Full-body workouts help improve overall body balance and coordination.

3. Calorie Burn: Engaging more muscles means burning more calories, which is essential for weight loss.

Seated Full-Body Exercises

1. Seated Knee Extensions: While seated, extend one leg straight in front of you, engaging your thigh muscles. Switch to the opposite leg after holding for a few breaths.

2. Seated Leg Lifts: Sit at the edge of your chair, lift both legs together, and hold them in the air. This strengthens your core and leg muscles.

3. Seated Torso Twist: Sit up straight and twist your torso to one side, using your core muscles. Do the same on the other side after returning back to the center.

4. Seated Rowing Motion: Hold your hands in front of you as if you're rowing a boat. Pull your elbows back and after that, then squeeze your shoulder blades together.

5. Seated Arm Circles: Extend your arms to the sides and make small circles. This works your shoulder muscles and enhances mobility.

6. Seated Marching: Sit with your feet flat on the floor. Lift one knee toward your chest and then lower it. Alternate between legs as if you're marching in place.

These seated full-body exercises are like the ingredients of a healthy recipe. When combined with regular Chair Yoga practice, they form a complete fitness regimen. Embrace the beauty of full-body workouts while seated, and you'll be amazed at the progress you make on your weight loss journey. Keep moving, keep engaging, and enjoy the journey toward a healthier you.

Advanced balance and flexibility exercises

In your Chair Yoga journey for weight loss, advancing your balance and flexibility is a key milestone. These advanced exercises are like the intricate brushstrokes of a skilled artist, adding depth and precision to your practice. Let's explore how you can enhance your balance and flexibility while staying comfortably seated.

1. Eagle Pose Variation:

   - Cross your right thigh over your left, like twisting a rope.

   - Lift your arms, bend your elbows, and bring your palms together.

   - This pose challenges your balance and enhances flexibility in your legs and shoulders.

2. King Pigeon Pose Variation:

   - Sit up straight and extend your right leg.

   - Bend your left knee, bringing your foot towards your hip.

   - Reach your arms back and clasp your hands.

   - This pose deepens the flexibility in your hips, back, and shoulders.

3. Seated Forward Fold with One Leg Extended:

   - Sit with your legs extended.

   - Bend one knee and bring the sole of your foot against your inner thigh.

   - Reach toward your extended foot.

   - This exercise increases flexibility in your hamstrings and improves balance.

4. Seated Spinal Twist with Leg Lift:

   - Sit up straight then place your right ankle on top of your left knee.

   - Turn your upper body to the right.

   - Lift your extended left leg.

   - This pose enhances spinal flexibility and challenges your balance.

5. Tree Pose Variation:

   - Lift your right leg and place your foot against your left calf or thigh.

   - Put your hands together at your chest.

   - This exercise improves balance and flexibility in your hips and legs.

6. Warrior III Pose Variation:

   - Extend one leg straight behind you while leaning forward.

- Raise your arms in front of you to help with balance.

- This pose enhances your balance and leg flexibility.

7. Seated Lotus Pose:
   - Sit with your legs crossed, bringing your feet onto your opposite thighs.
   - This is an advanced variation of the traditional Lotus Pose.
   - It deepens flexibility in your hips and legs.

8. Seated Boat Pose Variation:
   - Sit while bending your knees and your feet flat on the ground.
   - Raise one leg and then extend it forward.
   - Hold the pose and then switch legs.
   - This exercise strengthens your core and challenges balance.

Advanced balance and flexibility exercises are like refining a piece of art; each movement brings you closer to your masterpiece. As you practice these exercises regularly, you'll notice an increased sense of balance and greater flexibility in your body. These exercises are not only beneficial for weight loss but also for overall well-being. Keep painting your masterpiece, one brushstroke at a time, and watch your Chair Yoga practice transform.

Day 22: Celebrating Progress

Welcome to Day 22 of your Chair Yoga journey for weight loss. Today is a special day dedicated to "Celebrating Progress." Just as milestones mark significant moments in life, this day is all about recognizing how far you've come on your journey to a healthier and happier you.

Reflecting on Your Achievements

Look back on your adventure to this point for a moment. Think about the challenges you've faced and overcome, the poses you've mastered, and the consistency you've maintained. These are like the chapters of your success story.

Recognizing Small Victories

Celebrating progress is not just about reaching the destination; it's also about appreciating the small victories along the way. It's like finding joy in the little details of a beautiful painting.

Setting New Goals

As you celebrate progress, it's also a great time to set new goals. What would you like to achieve in the remaining days of your 28-day journey? Setting new goals is like charting your course on a map – it gives you direction and purpose.

Expressing Gratitude

Express gratitude for your journey. Gratitude is like the paint that adds richness and depth to your life's canvas. Be thankful for the opportunity to improve your health and well-being through Chair Yoga.

Mindful Celebrations

Incorporate mindfulness into your celebrations. Just as a connoisseur savors each bite of a delicious meal, savor every moment of your progress. Mindful celebrations can make your achievements even more fulfilling.

Sharing Your Journey

Consider sharing your progress with others. Whether it's with a friend, family member, or an online community, sharing your experiences can provide you with valuable support and encouragement, much like celebrating with loved ones.

Day 22 is Your Day

Day 22 is your day to celebrate the remarkable progress you've made on your Chair Yoga journey. It's like standing on a mountaintop, looking back at the path you've traveled, and feeling a deep sense of accomplishment.

As you continue your journey, remember that progress is not always measured in pounds or inches. It's about feeling stronger, more balanced, and healthier. Celebrate each step you take, and let the joy of your progress fuel your motivation for the days to come. Day 22 is a reminder that your Chair Yoga journey is a remarkable story, and you are the resilient, determined protagonist. Keep celebrating and keep moving forward – you're doing wonderfully!

Recognizing achievements and milestones

In your Chair Yoga journey for weight loss, recognizing your achievements and milestones is like marking the trail on a long hike. It keeps you motivated and reminds you of how far you've come. Let's explore the importance of acknowledging your progress and celebrating the milestones along the way.

Why It Matters

1. Motivation: Recognizing your achievements is like having a cheerleader on your side. It can boost your motivation when you see how far you've come.

2. Accountability: It holds you accountable for your journey, like a map guiding you to your destination.

3. Inspiration: Celebrating milestones can inspire you to set new goals and reach even higher, like a hiker spotting a new peak after conquering one.

How to Recognize Achievements and Milestones

1. Keep a Journal: Maintain a Chair Yoga journal to document your daily progress. Write about your practice, how you felt, and any improvements you've noticed. This is like leaving markers on the trail to show where you've been.

2. Take Photos: Visual progress can be motivating. Periodically take photos of yourself to see physical changes over time, much like taking snapshots of breathtaking scenery along your hike.

3. Use Technology: There are many apps and fitness trackers that can help you log your Chair Yoga practice and monitor your progress. These are like modern-day compasses to keep you on track.

Setting Milestones

1. Small Goals: Just as a hiker aims to reach a specific spot on the trail, set small, achievable goals in your Chair Yoga practice. Whether it's mastering a new pose or maintaining a consistent routine, these milestones add purpose to your journey.

2. Measurement: Make your milestones quantifiable. For example, set a goal to increase your flexibility, practice a certain pose, or stick to your Chair Yoga routine for a specific number of days. This is like measuring the distance you've covered.

3. Celebrate Progress: When you reach a milestone, celebrate it! It's like reaching a beautiful overlook on your hike – take a moment to soak it in and acknowledge your accomplishment.

The Journey Continues

Recognizing your achievements and milestones is not the end of your journey; it's a way to celebrate how far you've come and to fuel your motivation for the road ahead. Just like marking your trail with milestones, it gives you a sense of direction and purpose.

Your Chair Yoga journey is a story of growth, determination, and transformation. By recognizing your achievements and celebrating your milestones, you are crafting a beautiful narrative filled with success and personal triumphs. Keep moving forward with your head held high, and remember that every step you take is an achievement worth celebrating.

Daily tips for overcoming plateaus and self-care

In your Chair Yoga journey for weight loss, you may encounter plateaus where progress seems to stall. Just like a river that encounters a still pool before continuing its course, these plateaus are a natural part of the journey. Here are some daily tips to help you overcome plateaus and practice self-care.

Tip 1: Patience is Key

When progress slows, remember that patience is your best friend. It's like waiting for a flower to bloom – the process takes time. Be patient with yourself, and trust that change is happening, even if it's not immediately visible.

Tip 2: Mix It Up

If you find yourself doing the same routine every day, it might be time to mix things up. Try different Chair Yoga poses or explore new variations. Change is like a fresh breeze that revitalizes your journey.

Tip 3: Self-Care

Take time for self-care. Just as a hiker needs rest to recharge, you need moments of relaxation. Treat yourself to a warm bath, a good book, or a calming meditation. Self-care is like nourishment for your soul.

Tip 4: Listen to Your Body

Your body is like a compass; it knows the way. Listen to it. If you're feeling fatigued or sore, it's okay to take a break. This journey is a marathon and not a sprint.; it's a marathon. Be kind to your body, and it will support you.

Tip 5: Stay Mindful

Mindfulness is a powerful tool for overcoming plateaus. Being mindful during your practice helps you focus on the present moment, like a hiker appreciating the beauty of nature. It can break through mental barriers and keep you on track.

Tip 6: Set Realistic Goals

Review your goals and ensure they are realistic. Sometimes, plateaus occur because we set expectations that are too ambitious. Adjust your goals if needed, so they're attainable and motivating.

Tip 7: Celebrate Small Wins

Just as a hiker celebrates each new vista, celebrate your small wins. Did you hold a pose for an extra five seconds? Did you find a deeper level of relaxation? Celebrate these victories – they add up over time.

Tip 8: Seek Support

If you're feeling stuck, consider seeking support. Whether it's from a Chair Yoga instructor, a friend, or an online community, sharing your experiences can provide you with valuable insights and motivation.

Tip 9: Keep Moving Forward

Even on plateaus, keep moving forward. Just as a river slowly erodes rocks over time, your consistent efforts will lead to progress. Have faith in the process and remain dedicated to your journey.

Remember that overcoming plateaus is a normal part of any journey, and it's an opportunity for personal growth. By practicing self-care and implementing these tips, you can navigate through plateaus with grace and resilience. Your Chair Yoga journey for weight loss is an ongoing adventure, and each day is a chance to take a step closer to your goals. Keep moving forward with determination and self-compassion. You've got this!

Chapter 5: Week 4 - The Final Push

Welcome to Week 4 of your Chair Yoga journey for weight loss. It's time for "The Final Push." This week is like the climax of your favorite movie, where the hero faces their greatest challenges before reaching their goal. You're now in the home stretch, and the finish line is within sight.

Building on Your Progress

In the previous weeks, you've built a strong foundation, increased your mobility, and explored advanced poses. This week, you'll continue building on that progress, taking your practice to new heights.

Pushing Your Limits

Just as athletes push their limits in the final moments of a race, this week is about pushing your boundaries in Chair Yoga. You'll encounter more challenging poses and routines that will test your strength and determination.

Staying Consistent

Consistency is key as you enter "The Final Push." It's like the steady rhythm of a drumbeat that keeps you moving forward. Stick to your daily practice, and you'll see the rewards.

Setting Your Sights on Success

The finish line is in view, and it's time to set your sights on success. Your goal of weight loss is within reach, and the determination you've built will carry you through.

Daily Tips for Guidance

As always, our daily tips will be there to guide you through this crucial week. They'll provide you with the support and motivation you need, much like a trusted friend cheering you on during a challenging race.

Reflection and Celebration

In the midst of "The Final Push," don't forget to take a moment to reflect on your journey. Acknowledge and celebrate your accomplishments and progress. It's like taking a deep breath after running the final mile.

You're the Hero of Your Story

As you enter "The Final Push," remember that you are the hero of your own story. You've overcome challenges, pushed your limits, and remained consistent. This week is about bringing your journey to a triumphant conclusion.

With determination and the support of your daily tips, you'll make it to the finish line. Your Chair Yoga journey for weight loss is a remarkable story, and you're the resilient, determined protagonist. Keep pushing, keep believing, and keep moving forward – you're on the cusp of achieving your goal. The final chapter awaits, and it's a testament to your strength and dedication. Let's finish this journey strong!

Day 23-28: 28-Day Challenge Climax

Welcome to the grand finale of your Chair Yoga journey for weight loss – Day 23-28, the 28-Day Challenge Climax. Just as an epic story reaches its climax, these days are the culmination of your hard work, dedication, and determination. You're about to experience the sweet taste of success.

Day 23: Unleashing Your Inner Strength

As you embark on Day 23, it's like a superhero discovering their true powers. You'll push your boundaries, unleash your inner strength, and explore Chair Yoga poses that seemed impossible at the beginning.

Day 24: Deepening Your Mindfulness

Day 24 is all about deepening your mindfulness. It's similar to revealing the core of an onion by removing its layers. You'll connect with your breath, find stillness, and enhance your mental focus.

Day 25: Building Resilience

Resilience is your greatest ally on Day 25. It's like a rock standing strong against crashing waves. You'll face challenges, but your determination and resilience will see you through.

Day 26: Celebrating Progress

Day 26 is a day for celebrating progress. Like fireworks lighting up the night sky, you'll look back at your journey, recognizing how far you've come. It's a moment of reflection and celebration.

Day 27: Embracing the Present Moment

Day 27 is all about embracing the present moment. It's like catching a shooting star – a rare and beautiful occurrence. You'll stay mindful, fully experiencing each pose and breath.

Day 28: Victory and New Beginnings

Day 28 marks your victory and new beginnings. It's like completing a marathon and crossing the finish line. You've achieved your goal of completing the 28-Day Challenge, and it's a moment of triumph.

What Lies Ahead

As you reach the 28-Day Challenge Climax, remember that your Chair Yoga journey is not ending; it's evolving. Just as one chapter leads to the next, this accomplishment is the foundation for your ongoing health and wellness.

Your journey is a testament to your determination, resilience, and strength. With the support of your daily tips and the knowledge that you've reached the climax of your challenge, you're prepared for the next chapters of your story. As you continue to practice Chair Yoga, your health and well-being will flourish, and the journey will continue to be a remarkable adventure. Congratulations on reaching this remarkable milestone!

High-intensity chair yoga routines

In your Chair Yoga journey for weight loss, you might be wondering how to add intensity to your practice without leaving your chair. Just as a campfire's flames can dance higher, you can increase the intensity of your Chair Yoga routines. Here's how:

Why High-Intensity Chair Yoga?

High-intensity Chair Yoga is like adding more color to a painting – it brings depth and vibrancy to your practice. It can help you burn more calories, boost your heart rate, and improve your overall fitness.

Key Elements of High-Intensity Chair Yoga:

1. Faster Paced Sequences: Speed up the pace of your Chair Yoga routines. Just as a river flows faster in some parts, you can create sequences that are more dynamic and challenging.

2. Incorporate Strength Training: Add resistance bands or hand weights to your practice. This is like adding weights to a workout – it increases the intensity and helps build strength.

3. Interval Training: Alternate between bursts of high-intensity movements and moments of recovery. Interval training is like the ebb and flow of waves on a beach, and it can elevate your heart rate.

4. Jumpstart Your Heart: High knees, seated jumping jacks, and seated jogging can provide a cardiovascular workout. These exercises elevate your heart rate and are similar to brisk walking or light jogging.

5. Dynamic Chair Poses: Modify Chair Yoga poses to make them more challenging. For example, a high lunge with leg lifts or a seated mountain climber pose adds intensity to your practice.

Benefits of High-Intensity Chair Yoga:

1. Increased Calorie Burn: Just as a bonfire radiates more warmth, high-intensity Chair Yoga can help you burn more calories, supporting your weight loss goals.

2. Improved Cardiovascular Health: Elevating your heart rate in a safe and controlled manner can enhance your cardiovascular fitness.

3. Enhanced Strength and Endurance: High-intensity movements can strengthen your muscles and boost your endurance, helping you perform daily activities more easily.

Remember: Safety First

Before diving into high-intensity Chair Yoga, consult with your healthcare provider, especially if you have any medical conditions. Safety is paramount, and it's essential to perform high-intensity exercises with proper form to prevent injury.

High-intensity Chair Yoga is like adding a burst of energy to your practice, and it can be a fantastic way to advance your weight loss journey. Just as a dance performance crescendos with intensity, your Chair Yoga practice can become a dynamic, powerful, and effective way to reach your fitness goals. So, ignite the flames of high-intensity Chair Yoga and let your practice shine brightly!

Focusing on weight loss goals

In your Chair Yoga journey for weight loss, setting and focusing on your goals is like charting a course for a journey. It provides direction and purpose to your practice, much like a map guides a traveler. Here's how you can focus on your weight loss goals:

Define Your Goals Clearly

Just as a hiker plans their route, start by defining your weight loss goals clearly. Do you want to shed a certain number of pounds, feel more energetic, or fit into a specific clothing size? Your goals are like the destination on your journey, and having a clear endpoint makes the path more visible.

Break Goals into Smaller Steps

Breaking your goals into smaller, manageable steps is like dividing a long trail into sections. It makes the journey less overwhelming. For example, you can set weekly or monthly targets for weight loss, making the process feel achievable.

Measure Your Progress

Measuring your progress is like using markers along a trail to track your movement. Regularly weigh yourself, take measurements, or monitor how your clothes fit. These indicators provide evidence of your progress and help keep you motivated.

Stay Consistent

Consistency in your Chair Yoga practice is like the steady rhythm of footsteps on a path. Stick to your routine, and you'll steadily progress toward your goals. Regular practice is key to success.

Adjust Your Goals When Needed

Just as a traveler might change their course in response to obstacles, be willing to adjust your weight loss goals if necessary. Life can throw unexpected challenges, so flexibility is essential. Adapt your goals to your circumstances without losing sight of your destination.

Use Daily Tips for Guidance

Our daily tips are like signposts along your journey, providing guidance and support. They offer practical advice, motivation, and reminders to help you stay on track.

Celebrate Your Achievements

Celebrating your achievements is like pausing to admire a beautiful view on your journey. No matter how small, it's important to acknowledge your success. Celebrating success motivates you to keep moving forward.

Mindful Practice

Mindfulness in your Chair Yoga practice is like savoring the moment on your journey. It helps you stay focused on your goals and be aware of your body and its needs.

Stay Committed

Commitment is like the determination of a traveler to reach their destination. Regardless of challenges or setbacks, keep your commitment to your weight loss goals. Have confidence in your own abilities and potential for success.

Focusing on your weight loss goals in your Chair Yoga journey is like having a lighthouse guiding your way. With dedication and regular practice, you'll steadily progress toward your destination. Stay committed, be patient, and keep your goals in clear view. Your journey is a path to a healthier, happier you, and every step brings you closer to your destination.

Day 29: Reflecting on the Journey

Welcome to Day 29 of your Chair Yoga journey for weight loss. Today is a day of reflection, much like looking back at a well-trodden path. It's an opportunity to take stock of your incredible journey and celebrate how far you've come.

Why Reflect on the Journey?

Reflection is like a magnifying glass, helping you see your progress in finer detail. It's essential to look back at where you started, appreciate your achievements, and learn from your experiences.

What to Reflect On

1. Your Physical Progress: Reflect on how your body has changed throughout this journey. Have you become more flexible, gained strength, or noticed changes in your weight or measurements?

2. Mental and Emotional Growth: Consider how your mental and emotional well-being has evolved. Are you feeling more relaxed, focused, and in control of your thoughts and emotions?

3. Consistency: Think about your consistency in practicing Chair Yoga. How many days did you practice, and what motivated you to keep going?

4. Challenges and Breakthroughs: Recall the challenges you faced and the moments when you broke through them. These are like stepping stones that paved your path to progress.

5. Achieving Your Goals: Reflect on your weight loss goals. Have you achieved what you set out to accomplish, or are you well on your way to reaching them?

Expressing Gratitude

Take a moment to express gratitude for this incredible journey. Just as a traveler appreciates a warm meal after a long hike, be thankful for the opportunity to improve your health and well-being through Chair Yoga.

Planning the Next Steps

While Day 29 is about reflection, it's also a day to look ahead. What are your goals for the future? How will you continue your Chair Yoga practice? Plan your next steps and set new objectives.

Celebrating Your Achievements

Day 29 is like a victory lap at the end of a race. Celebrate your accomplishments, regardless of their size. These are the milestones that have made your journey remarkable.

Sharing Your Journey

Consider sharing your journey with others. Just as a storyteller shares their adventures, your experiences can inspire and encourage those around you. You never know who might be inspired by your dedication and determination.

A Remarkable Journey

Your Chair Yoga journey for weight loss has been nothing short of remarkable. It's a story of personal growth, resilience, and determination. As you reflect on Day 29, remember that every

Chair Yoga session was a step forward, every challenge was an opportunity for growth, and every moment was a chance to become a healthier and happier you.

Continue to embrace your journey with open arms, and let reflection be a guiding light as you move forward. Whether you're celebrating milestones or setting new goals, Day 29 is a testament to your strength and perseverance. Your Chair Yoga journey is an ongoing adventure, and the pages of your story continue to turn. Keep reflecting, keep growing, and keep reaching for the stars!

Self-assessment and future plans

In your Chair Yoga journey for weight loss, self-assessment is like looking in a mirror to understand where you are and where you're headed. As you near the end of this incredible journey, it's a valuable moment to evaluate your progress and make plans for the future.

Assessing Your Journey

1. Physical Progress: Take a look at the physical changes you've experienced. Have you become more flexible, toned, or noticed changes in your body? Assess your weight loss journey and how your body has transformed.

2. Mental and Emotional Well-Being: Consider how your mental and emotional health has improved. Are you feeling calmer, more focused, and in control of your thoughts and emotions? Reflect on the impact of Chair Yoga on your mental well-being.

3. Consistency and Commitment: Examine your consistency in practicing Chair Yoga. How many days did you practice, and what kept you motivated? Acknowledge your dedication and commitment to the journey.

4. Challenges and Breakthroughs: Reflect on the challenges you faced and how you overcame them. What were your most significant breakthroughs, and how did they impact your journey?

Setting Future Goals

1. Reevaluating Goals: Take time to reevaluate your weight loss goals. Are they still aligned with your aspirations, or do they need adjustment? Setting realistic goals is essential for continued progress.

2. Next Steps: What are your plans for the future of your Chair Yoga practice? Will you continue your daily routine, explore new variations, or seek more advanced Chair Yoga practices?

3. Nutrition and Diet: Consider how nutrition plays a role in your weight loss journey. Are there changes you'd like to make in your diet to support your goals?

4. Mindful Lifestyle: Integrate mindfulness into your daily life, not just during your Chair Yoga sessions. How can you be more mindful in your eating habits and everyday activities?

Expressing Gratitude

Just as a traveler appreciates a warm meal after a long hike, be thankful for the opportunity to improve your health and well-being through Chair Yoga.

Sharing Your Experience

Consider sharing your Chair Yoga journey with others. Just as a storyteller shares their adventures, your experiences can inspire and encourage those around you. Your journey is a source of motivation for those who may be considering a similar path.

A Continuing Adventure

Your Chair Yoga journey for weight loss is not merely a chapter; it's an ongoing adventure. Self-assessment and future planning are essential elements of this journey. Just as a ship's captain plots the course for the next leg of a voyage, you are steering your health and well-being toward new horizons.

Every day you practice Chair Yoga is a step forward in your remarkable story. Use self-assessment as your compass and future planning as your roadmap. With dedication and a clear vision, you'll continue to experience the benefits of Chair Yoga and journey toward a healthier and happier you. Keep assessing, keep planning, and keep moving forward!

Gradual transition to a balanced post-challenge routine

As you approach the end of your Chair Yoga journey for weight loss, it's essential to plan your transition into a balanced post-challenge routine. Just as a ship transitions from the excitement of a voyage to the steadiness of port, your routine should evolve with care and balance. Here's how to make the transition:

Acknowledge Your Achievements

Before transitioning, take time to acknowledge your accomplishments during the challenge. Reflect on how far you've come, the hurdles you've conquered, and the progress you've made toward your weight loss goals. Celebrate your achievements.

Setting Realistic Expectations

Understand that the post-challenge routine will be different from the intensity of the challenge itself. The challenge was like a sprint, and now it's time to settle into a steady jog. Set realistic expectations for your daily practice and fitness goals.

Maintain Chair Yoga Practice

While you may not continue with the same rigorous challenge routine, it's important to maintain your Chair Yoga practice. Consistency is key to long-term success. Design a balanced routine that includes regular Chair Yoga sessions, focusing on flexibility, strength, and mindfulness.

Incorporate Other Activities

Consider incorporating other physical activities into your routine. This is like adding variety to your diet to ensure you get a wide range of nutrients. Explore gentle walks, swimming, or other low-impact exercises to complement your Chair Yoga practice.

Mindful Eating and Balanced Diet

Just as Chair Yoga enhances mindfulness, continue to be mindful of your eating habits. A balanced diet is essential for maintaining your weight loss. Ensure that you're eating a variety of nutrient-rich foods, practicing portion control, and staying hydrated.

Self-Care and Recovery

Integrate self-care into your daily routine. Prioritize relaxation, get enough sleep, and manage stress. Self-care is like the wind in your sails; it provides energy for the journey ahead.

Regular Self-Assessment

Continue to self-assess regularly. Just as a sailor checks the condition of the ship, periodically evaluate your progress, adjust your goals, and make necessary changes to your routine.

Stay Connected and Share Your Journey

Stay connected with the Chair Yoga community and share your post-challenge experiences. Your journey is like a map for others, and your insights and encouragement can inspire and support fellow practitioners.

Celebrate Your Journey

Remember that this transition is not an end but a continuation of your remarkable journey. Celebrate your past achievements and be excited about the path that lies ahead.

A Lifelong Adventure

Your Chair Yoga journey is not just a challenge; it's a lifelong adventure. As you transition into a balanced post-challenge routine, keep in mind that your health and well-being are ongoing pursuits. By maintaining a balanced and sustainable routine, you'll continue to reap the benefits of Chair Yoga and work toward a healthier and happier you. Keep balancing, keep evolving, and keep enjoying the journey!

Conclusion

Dear Reader,

As we conclude this extraordinary journey on "Chair Yoga for Weight Loss," it's a moment to reflect on the journey you've undertaken, the stories you've discovered, and the knowledge you've gained. In this concluding chapter, we'll explore success stories and transformations, offer encouragement for a lifelong Chair Yoga practice, and share our final thoughts on achieving balance, flexibility, and weight loss through Chair Yoga.

Success Stories and Transformations

Throughout your journey, you've undoubtedly encountered success stories and transformations from individuals who have embraced Chair Yoga for weight loss. Their stories are like guiding stars, showing you what's possible. Remember that their achievements are a testament to the power of consistency, determination, and the practice of Chair Yoga. As you read these stories, take inspiration from those who have walked this path before you. Their journeys are a testament to the transformative potential of Chair Yoga.

Encouragement for a Lifelong Chair Yoga Practice

Chair Yoga is not just a 28-day challenge; it's a lifelong practice. It's a journey of health, wellness, and self-discovery that continues beyond the pages of this book. We encourage you to keep the flame of your practice alive, to make Chair Yoga a part of your daily routine, and to explore the benefits it can bring to your life.

Final Thoughts on Achieving Balance, Flexibility, and Weight Loss Through Chair Yoga

In these final thoughts, we want to emphasize the importance of balance in your Chair Yoga practice. Balance is not only about the physical poses but also about integrating mindfulness into your daily life. It's about achieving a sense of equilibrium, both in your body and mind. As you embark on a lifelong Chair Yoga journey, keep in mind that flexibility and weight loss are not just goals but ongoing processes. The practice of Chair Yoga is a tool that can support your goals while also enhancing your overall well-being.

A New Beginning

As you close the pages of this book, remember that it's not the end of your Chair Yoga journey; it's a new beginning. You have so much more to write in the chapters that lie ahead of you in your story. Your journey is not just about weight loss; it's about a lifelong commitment to health, happiness, and self-care.

Stay Connected and Keep Sharing

We encourage you to stay connected with the Chair Yoga community, share your experiences, and inspire others with your journey. Your story can be a source of motivation for fellow practitioners, and together, we can support one another in this ongoing adventure.

We are grateful that you have joined us on this adventure. As you continue to explore the world of Chair Yoga and all the benefits it can bring, remember that your story is remarkable, your path is unique, and your potential is boundless. Keep practicing, keep growing, and keep reaching for your goals. Your Chair Yoga journey is a lifelong adventure, and we're excited to continue it with you.

With warm regards and best wishes for your future,

Anthony D. Anderson,
Author of Chair Yoga for Weight Loss.